C000183518

Change the Way You Cook

Everyday Instant Pot Homemade Meals the Whole

Family Will Love

Shannon Robertson

© Copyright 2021 - All rights reserved.

The content contained within this book may not be reproduced, duplicated or transmitted without direct written permission from the author or the publisher.

Under no circumstances will any blame or legal responsibility be held against the publisher, or author, for any damages, reparation, or monetary loss due to the information contained within this book. Either directly or indirectly.

Legal Notice:

This book is copyright protected. This book is only for personal use. You cannot amend, distribute, sell, use, quote or paraphrase any part, or the content within this book, without the consent of the author or publisher.

Disclaimer Notice:

Please note the information contained within this document is for educational and entertainment purposes only. All effort has been executed to present accurate, up to date, and reliable, complete information. No warranties of any kind are declared or implied. Readers acknowledge that the author is not engaging in the rendering of legal, financial, medical or professional advice. The content within this book has been derived from various sources. Please consult a licensed professional before attempting any techniques outlined in this book.

By reading this document, the reader agrees that under no circumstances is the author responsible for any losses, direct or indirect, which are incurred as a result of the use of information contained within this document, including, but not limited to, — errors, omissions, or inaccuracies.

Sommario

Introduction..8

Desserts...10

Pineapple Fluffy Cake..10

Vanilla Strawberry Cheesecake..14

Keto Cinnamon Donuts...18

Chocolate Lava Cups...22

Applesauce..26

Dark Chocolate Sauce..29

Vanilla Apple Cake...32

Frozen Blueberry Muffins...36

Cinnamon Pumpkin Cake...39

Strawberry Pie..43

Lemon Flan...46

Natural Ice Cream..50

Almond Vanilla Shake.......................................53

Cocoa Muffins..56

Cardamom Pudding...60

Chocolate Bacon..64

Lemon Curd..66

Lime Coconut Pie...69

Coconut Blondies...73

Hot Baked Apples...76

Vanilla Pumpkin Pudding 79

Grated Nutmeg Pie..83

Condensed Cream...87

Crème Brule 90

Coconut Macaroons..93

Vanilla Bars..96

Avocado and Coconut Mousse 99

Ricotta and Nutmeg Pie...103

Nutmeg Crumble..106

Blackberry Compote...109

Sponge Cake..112

Zucchini "Apple" Baked Crisp 115

Conclusion...119

Introduction

This total as well as beneficial overview to instant pot cooking with over 1000 dishes for morning meal, dinner, dinner, and also treats! This is among the most comprehensive split second pot cookbooks ever published thanks to its selection and accurate guidelines. Cutting-edge recipes as well as standards, contemporary take on family members's most enjoyed meals-- all this is tasty, easy and also naturally as healthy as it can be. Adjustment the method you prepare with these ingenious split second pot instructions. Required a brand-new dinner or a treat? Here you are! Ideal instant pot dishes integrated in a couple of easy steps, even a newbie can do it! The instantaneous pot specifies the method you cook everyday. This immediate pot recipe book aids you make the outright most out of your regular menu. The only instant pot book you will ever before require with the best collection of recipes will help you towards a simpler and healthier kitchen experience. If you want to save time cooking dishes extra effectively, if you intend to supply your household food that can

please even the pickiest eater, you are in the appropriate area!

Master your immediate pot and also make your cooking needs suit

your busy way of life.

Desserts

Pineapple Fluffy Cake

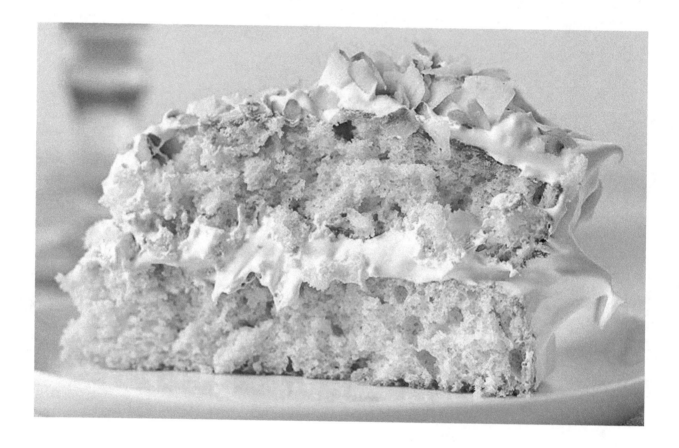

Prep time: 15 minutes

Cooking time: 30 minutes

Servings: 10

Ingredients

- 9 ounces pineapple, canned

- 4 eggs

- 1 cup almond flour

- 1 cup sour cream

- 1 teaspoon baking soda

- 1 tablespoon lemon juice

- 1 teaspoon cinnamon

- ½ cup erythritol

- 2 tablespoons butter

Directions:

1. Beat the eggs in the mixing bowl and whisk them with the help of the whisker.

2. After this, add sour cream and continue to whisk the mixture for 1 minute more.

3. Then add baking soda and lemon juice. Stir the mixture gently.

4. Then add Erythritol, cinnamon, butter, and almond flour. Mix the mixture up with the help of the hand mixer for 5 minutes.

5. Then chop the canned pineapples and add them to the dough. Mix up the dough with the help of the spoon.

6. Then pour the dough in the pressure cooker and close the lid. Cook the dish at the manual mode for 30 minutes.

7. When the time is over – open the pressure cooker and check if the cake is cooked. Remove the cake from the pressure cooker and chill it well.

8. Slice the cake and serve. Enjoy!

Nutrition: calories 176, fat 14.2, fiber 1.7, carbs 16.7, protein 5.5

Vanilla Strawberry Cheesecake

Prep time: 10 minutes

Cooking time: 24 minutes

Servings: 6

Ingredients

- 1 cup strawberries

- 1 cup cream

- 2 eggs

- ½ cup Erythritol

- 7 ounces almond arrowroot crackers

- 5 tablespoon butter

- 1 teaspoon vanilla sugar

- ¼ teaspoon nutmeg

- 3 tablespoons low-fat caramel

Directions:

1. Crush the crackers well and combine them with the butter.

   Mix well until smooth. Beat the eggs in a mixing bowl.

2. Add the sugar, vanilla Erythritol, nutmeg, and cream. Whisk the mixture well. Wash the strawberries and slice them.

3. Put the cracker mixture in the pressure cooker and flatten it to make the crust. Pour the cream mixture into the crust and flatten it using a spoon.

4. Dip the sliced strawberries in the cream mixture and close the pressure cooker lid. Cook at "Pressure" mode for 24 minutes.

5. When the cooking time ends, remove the cheesecake from the pressure cooker carefully and chill it in the refrigerator.

6. Sprinkle the cheesecake with the caramel, cut into slices and serve.

Nutrition: calories 148, fat 13.4, fiber 0.5, carbs 21.2, protein 2.4

Keto Cinnamon Donuts

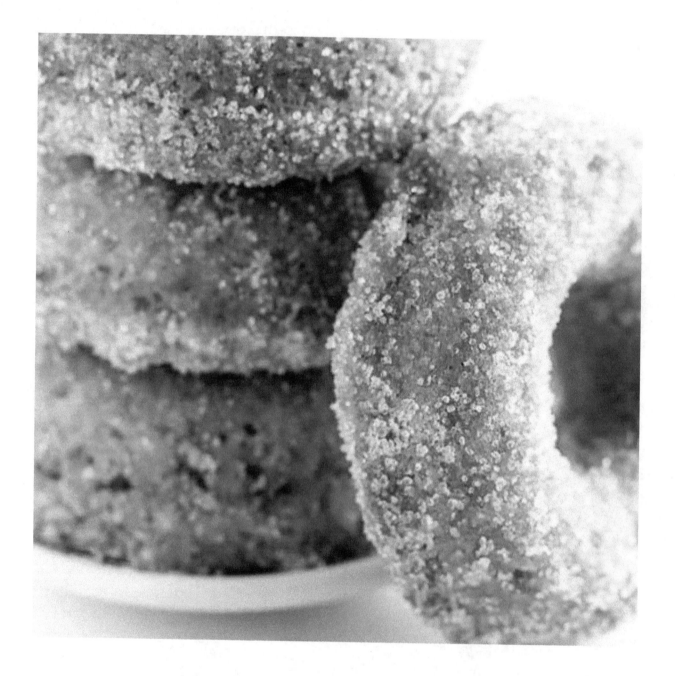

Prep time: 15 minutes

Cooking time: 6 minutes

Servings: 8

Ingredients

- 1 cup of coconut milk

- 3 eggs, beaten

- 1 teaspoon vanilla extract

- 1cup coconut flour

- ½ cup almond flour

- 1 teaspoon baking powder

- ½ cup Erythritol

- 1 tablespoon ground cinnamon

- 1 teaspoon olive oil

Directions:

1. Mix up together coconut milk, beaten eggs, vanilla extract, coconut flour, and almond flour. Add baking powder and olive oil.

2. Knead the non-sticky dough. Roll it up and make 8 donuts with the help of the cutter.

3. Place the donuts in the air fryer basket of Foodie and close the lid.

4. Cook the donuts at 355F for 3 minutes from each side. After this, mix up together Erythritol and ground cinnamon. Coat every cooked donut in the cinnamon mixture.

Nutrition: calories 204, fat 14.2, fiber 7.9, carbs 26.4, protein 6.3

Chocolate Lava Cups

Prep time: 10 minutes

Cooking time: 10 minutes

Servings: 4

Ingredients

- ½ cup Erythritol

- 3 whole eggs

- 1 cup coconut flour

- 1-ounce chocolate

- 4 egg yolks

- 1 teaspoon vanilla sugar

- 8 ounces butter

- 1 teaspoon instant coffee

Directions:

1. Beat the whole eggs in a mixing bowl.

2. Add the egg yolks and continue to whisk for a minute. Add the Erythritol and mix well using a hand mixer.

3. Melt the chocolate and butter. Add the melted chocolate to the egg mixture slowly. Add the coconut flour, instant coffee, and vanilla sugar.

4. Mix until smooth.

5. Pour the chocolate mixture into ramekins and place them in the pressure cooker trivet. Transfer the trivet in the pressure cooker.

6. Close the pressure cooker lid and set it to "Bake/Roast." Cook for 10 minutes.

7. When the cooking time ends, open the pressure cooker and remove the trivet. Let the ramekins cool for a few minutes and serve.

Nutrition: calories 644, fat 57.6, fiber 12.1, carbs 23.3, protein 11.6

Applesauce

Prep time: 10 minutes

Cooking time: 16 minutes

Servings: 5

Ingredients

- ½ pound apples

- 2 cup of water

- 1 teaspoon cinnamon

- 1 teaspoon Erythritol

Directions:

1. Wash the apples and peel them. Chop the apples and place them in the pressure cooker. Add the water and mix well.

2. Close the lid and cook the apples at "Pressure" for 16 minutes. Release the pressure and open the pressure cooker lid.

3. Transfer the cooked apples to a blender and blend well.

4. Add the cinnamon and Erythritol and blend for another minute until smooth.

5. Chill the applesauce in the refrigerator before serving.

Nutrition: calories 13, fat 0.1, fiber 0.8, carbs 3.5, protein 0.1

Dark Chocolate Sauce

Prep time: 5 minutes

Cooking time: 2 minutes

Servings: 4

Ingredients

- 1 tablespoon cocoa powder

- 4 tablespoons butter

- 1 oz dark chocolate

- 1 tablespoon Erythritol

Directions:

1. Place butter, cocoa powder, and dark chocolate in the Foodi Pressure cooker. Add Erythritol and stir gently.

2. Close the lid and cook the mixture on High-pressure mode for 2 minutes. Then make quick pressure release.

3. Open the lid and whisk the cooked mixture well.

4. Transfer it in the glass jar and store in the fridge up to 3 days.

Nutrition: calories 143, fat 13.8, fiber 0.6, carbs 8, protein 0.9

Vanilla Apple Cake

Prep time: 10 minutes

Cooking time: 18 minutes

Servings: 10

Ingredients

- 1 teaspoon cinnamon

- ½ cup Erythritol

- 1 cup coconut flour

- 1 egg

- 1 apple

- 1 cup sour cream

- 1 tablespoon vanilla sugar

- 1 teaspoon ground ginger

- 5 ounces butter

- 1 tablespoon orange juice

- 12 teaspoons lemon zest

Directions:

1. Beat the egg in the mixing bowl and whisk for a minute.

2. Add the coconut flour, sour cream, vanilla sugar, orange juice, and lemon zest. Mix until smooth. Remove the seeds from the apple and dice.

3. Sprinkle the chopped apple with Erythritol, cinnamon, and ground ginger. Mix well and combine it with the dough, mixing well.

4. Melt the butter and add it to the dough and stir well.

5. Add the apple dough in the pressure cooker. Close the lid and cook at "Pressure" for 18 minutes.

6. When the cooking time ends, open the pressure cooker lid and let the cake rest.

7. Remove the cake from the pressure cooker and transfer it to a serving plate. Slice it and serve.

Nutrition: calories 225, fat 18, fiber 5.6, carbs 23.9, protein 3.2

Frozen Blueberry Muffins

Prep time: 15 minutes

Cooking time: 10 minutes

Servings: 6

Ingredients

- 1 cup frozen blueberries

- 1 ½ cup coconut flour

- 1 teaspoon baking powder

- 1 tablespoon apple cider vinegar

- 1 tablespoon coconut

- ½ cup almond milk

- 2 eggs

- 1 teaspoon vanilla extract

- 1 teaspoon olive oil

Directions:

1. Place the coconut flour, baking soda, apple cider vinegar, coconut, almond milk, eggs, and vanilla extract in a food processor.

2. Blend the mixture well.

3. Add the frozen blueberries and blend the mixture for 30 seconds more. Take the muffin molds and fill half of every mold with the batter.

4. Place the muffins molds on the trivet and transfer it to the pressure cooker. Close the lid and cook at "Pressure" mode for 10 minutes.

5. When the muffins are baked, remove them from the pressure cooker. Let them rest and serve.

Nutrition: calories 214, fat 10.4, fiber 13.1, carbs 25.4, protein 6.5

Cinnamon Pumpkin Cake

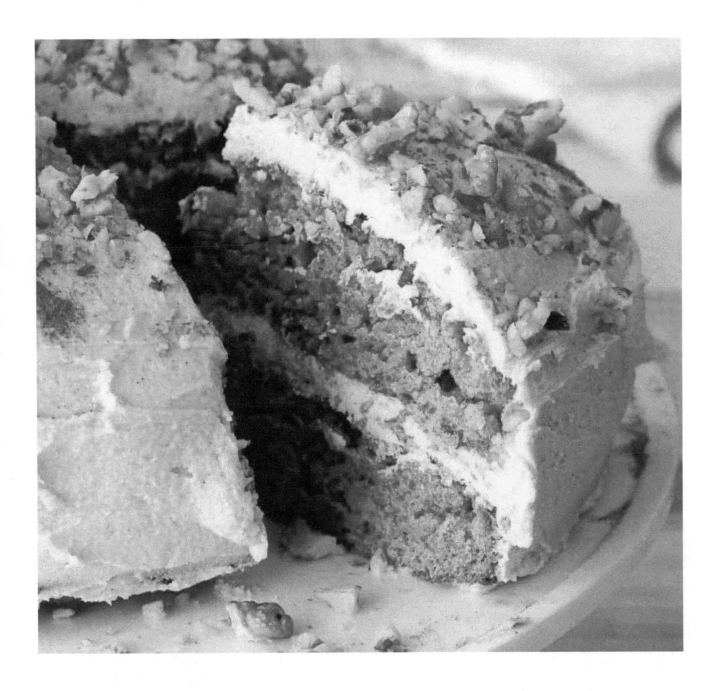

Prep time: 15 minutes

Cooking time: 25 minutes

Servings: 10

Ingredients

- 3 cups canned pumpkin

- 1 teaspoon cinnamon

- 3 cup coconut flour

- 2 eggs

- 1 tablespoon baking powder

- 1 tablespoon apple cider vinegar

- 1/3 cup Erythritol

- 1 teaspoon vanilla extract

- 1 teaspoon olive oil

- ½ cup walnuts

- 1 teaspoon salt

Directions:

1. Mash the canned pumpkin well. Combine the coconut flour, baking powder, apple cider vinegar, Erythritol, vanilla extract, and salt and stir well.

2. Beat the eggs in the separate bowl. Add the eggs to the coconut flour mixture and stir. Crush the walnuts.

3. Combine the mashed pumpkin and flour mixture together.

4. Knead the dough until smooth. Add crushed walnuts and knead the dough for another minute.

5. Spray the pressure cooker with olive oil. Add the pumpkin dough and flatten it into the shape of the cake.

6. Close the pressure cooker lid. Set at "Pressure" mode and cook the cake for 25 minutes. Check if the cake is cooked using a toothpick, and remove it from the pressure cooker. Let it rest, slice and serve.

Nutrition: calories 228, fat 8.9, fiber 17.1, carbs 31.6, protein 8.2

Strawberry Pie

Prep time: 15 minutes

Cooking time: 15 minutes

Servings: 4

Ingredients

- 1 cup almond flour

- 1/3 cup butter, softened

- 1 tablespoon swerve

- 1 teaspoon baking powder

- ¼ cup almond milk

- ¼ cup strawberries, sliced

Directions:

1. Make the batter: mix up together almond flour, softened butter, swerve, baking powder, and almond milk. Whisk it until smooth.

2. Pour the mixture in the Foodie. Place the sliced strawberries over the batter and press them gently to make the berry layer.

3. Close and seal the lid. Set High-pressure mode and cook pie for 15 minutes.

4. Then allow natural pressure release for 5 minutes. Chill the pie well and cut it into servings.

Nutrition: calories 214, fat 22.5, fiber 1.3, carbs 7.4, protein 2.1

Lemon Flan

Prep time: 15 minutes

Cooking time: 20 minutes

Servings: 4

Ingredients

- ¼ cup Erythritol

- 3 tablespoons water

- ½ cup coconut cream

- ½ cup cream

- 2 eggs

- ½ teaspoon salt

- 1 tablespoon lemon juice

- 1 teaspoon lemon zest

- 1 teaspoon vanilla extract

Directions:

1. Combine Erythritol and water together into the pressure cooker and preheat it at "Pressure" mode.

2. Stir the mixture continuously until smooth caramel forms. Pour the caramel into the ramekins. Set the pressure cooker to "Sauté" mode.

3. Pour the cream in the pressure cooker and cook it for 30 seconds. Beat the eggs in a mixing bowl.

4. Add the eggs slowly to the preheated cream, stirring constantly. Add the salt, lemon zest, vanilla extract, and coconut cream.

5. Add the lemon juice and mix well. Cook for 1 minute, stirring constantly. Pour the cream mixture into the ramekins.

6. Place the ramekins in the pressure cooker trivet and transfer it to the pressure cooker. Close the pressure cooker lid.

7. Cook for 8 minutes at "Pressure."

8. Remove the ramekins from the pressure cooker and chill them in the refrigerator for several hours before serving.

Nutrition: calories 181, fat 16.82, fiber 0.5, carbs 3.27, protein 5.12

Natural Ice Cream

Prep time: 10 minutes

Cooking time: 5 minutes

Servings: 4

Ingredients

- 1 cup heavy cream

- 4 egg yolks

- 3 teaspoons Erythritol

- 1 tablespoon vanilla extract

Directions:

1. Whisk together Erythritol and egg yolks. Then pour heavy cream in the Foodie.

2. Add egg yolk mixture and vanilla extract. Cook the liquid on High-pressure mode for 5 minutes.

3. Then make a quick pressure release and open the lid. Stir it well and transfer in the mixing bowl.

4. Mix up the mixture with the help of the hand mixer until it starts to be thick.

5. Then transfer it in the ice cream maker and make ice cream according to the directions of the manufacturer.

Nutrition: calories 365, fat 15.6, fiber 0, carbs 5.6, protein 3.3

Almond Vanilla Shake

Prep time: 10 minutes

Cooking time: 3 minutes

Servings: 3

Ingredients

- 1 cup almond milk

- 2 tablespoons swerve

- 1 teaspoon vanilla extract

- 1 tablespoon almond flour

- 2 tablespoons butter

- 1 tablespoon walnuts, chopped

Directions:

1. Pour almond milk in the Foodie. Add swerve and vanilla extract.

2. After this, add butter and close the lid.

3. Cook the liquid on High-pressure mode for 3 minutes.

4. Then allow natural pressure release for 10 minutes.

5. Add almond flour and mix up the liquid until smooth.

6. Add walnuts and stir gently. Pour the cooked cake in the serving glasses and serve warm.

Nutrition: calories 286, fat 29.4, fiber 2.2, carbs 8.7, protein 3

Cocoa Muffins

Prep time: 10 minutes

Cooking time: 10 minutes

Servings: 7

Ingredients

- 3 tablespoons cocoa

- ½ cup Erythritol

- 2 eggs

- 1 teaspoon baking soda

- 1 tablespoon lemon juice

- 1 cup coconut flour

- 1 cup plain yogurt

- ½ teaspoon salt

- 1 teaspoon olive oil

Directions:

1. Beat the eggs in a mixing bowl. Add the cocoa and mix well.

2. Combine the baking soda with the lemon juice and add to the egg mixture, mixing well. Add Erythritol and yogurt and mix again.

3. Add the salt and coconut flour.

4. Mix well using a hand mixer, until smooth batter forms. Spray the muffin forms with olive oil. Pour the batter into the muffin forms until halfway full.

5. Place the muffins forms in the pressure cooker.

6. Set to "Pressure" mode and close the lid. Cook the muffins for 10 minutes.

7. When the muffins are cooked, remove them from the pressure cooker. Let the muffins rest, then remove them from the muffin forms and serve.

Nutrition: calories 123, fat 4.4, fiber 7.6, carbs 29, protein 6.3

Cardamom Pudding

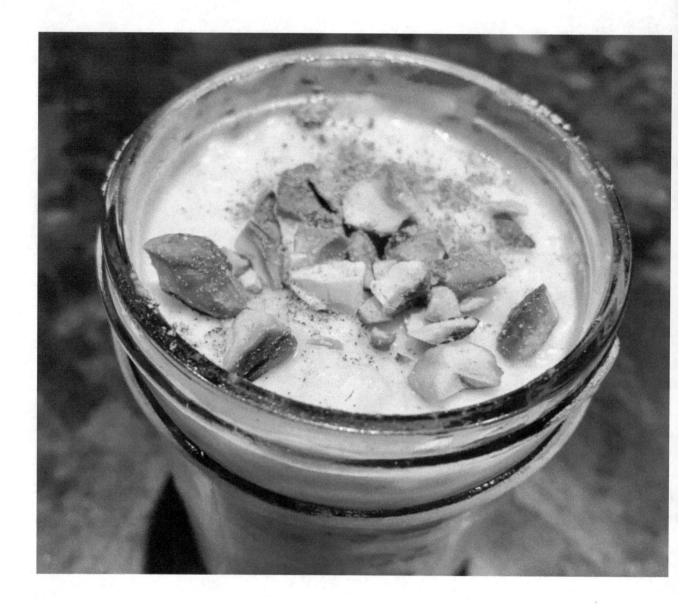

Prep time: 10 minutes

Cooking time: 21 minutes

Servings: 5

Ingredients

- 1 cup heavy cream

- ½ cup half and half

- 2 tablespoons starch

- 4 egg yolk

- 2 tablespoons Erythritol

- 1 teaspoon ground cardamom

- 1 teaspoon vanilla extract

Directions:

1. Whisk the heavy cream, then add the half and half and starch.

2. Whisk the mixture for another minute. Add egg yolks and use a hand mixer to combine the mixture.

3. Add Erythritol, ground cardamom, and vanilla extract. Mix well for another minute. Place the cream mixture in the glass form.

4. Put the trivet in the pressure cooker and add the glass form with the uncooked pudding. Close the pressure cooker lid cook at "Pressure" for 21 minutes.

5. Remove the pudding from the pressure cooker and chill in the refrigerator for a couple of hours before serving.

Nutrition: calories 175, fat 15.3, fiber 0.1, carbs 11, protein 3.4

Chocolate Bacon

Prep time: 10 minutes

Cooking time: 4 minutes

Servings: 6

Ingredients

- 6 bacon slices

- 2 oz dark chocolate, melted

Directions:

1. Place the bacon slices in the basket and close the lid.

2. Set the Air fryer mode and cook bacon for 4 minutes. Flip it onto another side after 2 minutes of cooking.

3. Then dip the cooked bacon in the melted chocolate and let it chill until the chocolate is solid.

Nutrition: calories 156, fat 11.3, fiber 0.5, carbs 4.1, protein 8

Lemon Curd

Prep time: 10 minutes

Cooking time: 13 minutes

Servings: 5

Ingredients

- 4 tablespoons butter

- ½ cup Erythritol

- 3 egg yolks

- 3 tablespoons lemon zest

- 1 cup lemon juice

- 1 teaspoon vanilla extract

Directions:

1. Place the butter in a blender and add Erythritol. Blend the mixture for 2 minutes.

2. Add the egg yolks and lemon zest. Blend the mixture for 3 minutes. Add the lemon juice and vanilla extract.

3. Blend for 30 seconds. Pour water in the pressure cooker and place the trivet inside. Pour the curd mixture into glass jars and transfer them in the pressure cooker.

4. Close the pressure cooker lid and cook the lemon curd on "Pressure" mode for 13 minutes.

5. When the lemon curd is cooked, release the pressure and remove the glass jars with the lemon curd from the pressure cooker.

6. For the best results, chill the lemon curd in the refrigerator for at least 8 hours.

Nutrition: calories 130, fat 12.3, fiber 0.4, carbs 2.3, protein 2.2

Lime Coconut Pie

Prep time: 30 minutes

Cooking time: 30 minutes

Servings: 12

Ingredients

- 1 teaspoon baking powder

- 1 cup whey

- 1 teaspoon salt

- 1 cup Erythritol

- 1 lime

- 1 teaspoon cinnamon

- 1 tablespoon butter

- 1 teaspoon cardamom

- 2 cups coconut flour

Directions:

1. Combine the baking powder, whey, and Erythritol in a mixing bowl. Mix well.

2. Add the coconut flour, cardamom, butter, cinnamon, and salt.

3. Mix well and knead the dough. Leave the dough in the bowl under the towel in the warm place for 10 minutes. Slice the limes.

4. Make the layer from the limes in the pressure cooker.

5. Pour the dough in the pressure cooker and flatten it. Close the pressure cooker lid and cook at "Pressure" for 20 minutes.

6. When the pie is cooked, open the pressure cooker lid and let the pie rest. Turn the pie onto a serving plate. Slice the pie and serve.

Nutrition: calories 96, fat 3, fiber 8.3, carbs 31.5, protein 2.9

Coconut Blondies

Prep time: 15 minutes

Cooking time: 10 minutes

Servings: 6

Ingredients

- 1 teaspoon baking powder

- 1 teaspoon lemon juice

- 4 tablespoons butter, softened

- 1 cup almond flour

- ¼ cup flax meal

- 3 tablespoons Erythritol

- 1 teaspoon vanilla extract

- 2 tablespoons coconut flakes

Directions:

1. In the mixing bowl mix up together all the ingredients and knead the smooth and non-sticky dough.

2. Place the dough in the Foodie and cut it into small bars.

3. Close the lid and cook on High-pressure mode for 10 minutes. Then allow natural pressure release for 10 minutes more.

4. Chill the cooked dessert well and transfer on the plate.

Nutrition: calories 123, fat 12.3, fiber 2, carbs 3.1, protein 2.2

Hot Baked Apples

Prep time: 10 minutes

Cooking time: 15 minutes

Servings: 5

Ingredients

- 5 red apples

- 1 tablespoon stevia, powdered

- ½ cup almonds

- 1 teaspoon cinnamon

- 1 cup of water

Directions:

1. Wash the apples and cut the tops off.

2. Remove the seeds and flesh from the apples to make apple cups. Crush the almonds. Sprinkle the apples with the cinnamon and stevia.

3. Fill the apples with the almond mixture and cover them with the apple tops.

4. Pour water in the pressure cooker.

5. Add the stuffed apples and close the pressure cooker lid. Cook the apples at "Sauté" mode for 15 minutes.

6. When the cooking time ends, transfer the apples to a serving plate.

Nutrition: calories 172, fat 5.2, fiber 6.8, carbs 33.2, protein 2.6

Vanilla Pumpkin Pudding

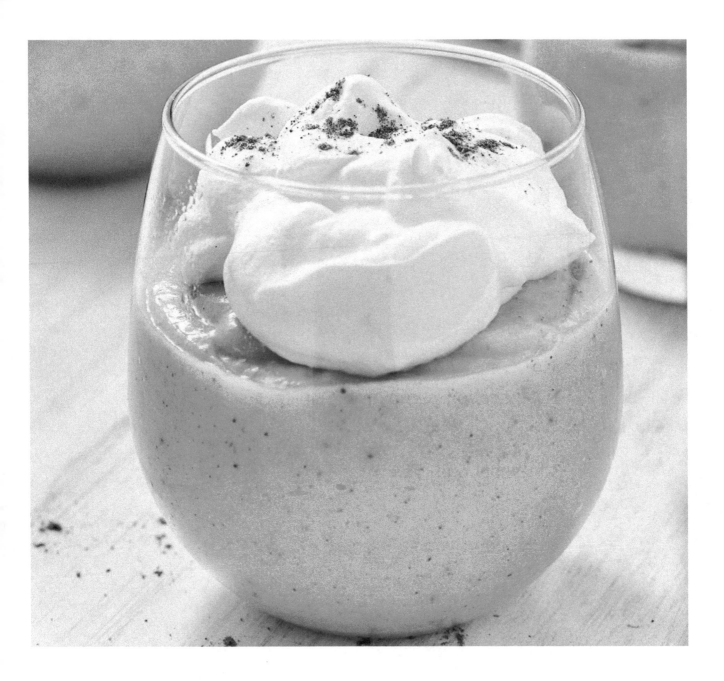

Prep time: 10 minutes

Cooking time: 35 minutes

Servings: 7

Ingredients

- 1 pound pumpkin

- 1 tablespoon pumpkin pie spice

- 3 tablespoons cream

- 1 teaspoon vanilla extract

- 4 cups of water

- 1 teaspoon butter

Directions:

1. Peel the pumpkin and chop it. Place the pumpkin in the pressure cooker and add water. Close the pressure cooker lid and cook at "Pressure" mode for 20 minutes.

2. Strain the pumpkin and mash it using a fork. Sprinkle the pumpkin with the pumpkin pie spices, vanilla extract, butter, and cream.

3. Mix well until smooth.

4. Pour the pumpkin mixture into a large ramekin, wrap it with aluminum foil, and place it in the pressure cooker trivet.

5. Pour the water in the pressure cooker, avoiding the ramekin.

6. Close the pressure cooker lid and cook at "Sauté" mode for 15 minutes.

7. Remove the pudding from the pressure cooker and let it rest. Remove the foil and serve.

Nutrition: calories 26, fat 1, fiber 0.8, carbs 4, protein 0.6

Grated Nutmeg Pie

Prep time: 25 minutes

Cooking time: 25 minutes

Servings: 7

Ingredients

- 1 cup strawberries, mashed

- 7 ounces butter

- 1 teaspoon salt

- 1 cup almond flour

- 1 teaspoon vanilla extract

- 1 tablespoon lemon zest

- 1 tablespoon turmeric

- 1 teaspoon nutmeg

- ½ teaspoon ground ginger

Directions:

1. Grate the butter in a mixing bowl.

2. Sprinkle it with the salt, vanilla extract, lemon zest, turmeric, nutmeg, and ground ginger. Sift the almond flour into the bowl and knead the dough using your hands.

3. Place the dough in the freezer for 15 minutes.

4. Remove the dough from the freezer and cut it in half. Grate the one part of the dough in the pressure cooker.

5. Sprinkle the grated dough with the strawberries. Flatten it well to make a layer. Grate the second part of the dough in the pressure cooker.

6. Close the lid and cook at "Pressure" mode for 25 minutes.

7. When the cooking time ends, transfer the pie to a serving plate and let it rest. Cut into slices and serve.

Nutrition: calories 309, fat 31.3, fiber 2.5, carbs 6.2, protein 3.9

Condensed Cream

Prep time: 10 minutes

Cooking time: 40 minutes

Servings: 7

Ingredients

- 3 cups cream

- 5 egg yolks

- 1 cup Erythritol

- 1 teaspoon vanilla extract

Directions:

1. Whisk the yolks in a mixing bowl.

2. Combine the cream and Erythritol together in the pressure cooker. Set the pressure cooker to "Sauté" mode.

3. Add the vanilla extract and cook for 10 minutes, stirring frequently. Mix the ingredients and add the egg yolks slowly and stir well.

4. Close the pressure cooker and cook at "Pressure" mode for 30 minutes.

5. When the cooking time ends, remove the milk and refrigerate immediately.

Nutrition: calories 106, fat 8.9, fiber 0, carbs 3.7, protein 2.8

Crème Brule

Prep time: 10 minutes

Cooking time: 20 minutes

Servings: 6

Ingredients

- 5 tablespoon Erythritol

- 2 cup cream

- ½ teaspoon salt

- 10 egg yolks

Directions:

1. Put the egg yolks in a mixing bowl and use a hand mixer to combine for a minute.

2. Add salt and continue to blend the egg mixture for another minute. When the mixture becomes fluffy, add cream. Mix well for another minute.

3. Sprinkle the glass ramekins with Erythritol and pour the cream mixture into each one. Pour the water in the pressure cooker and place the trivet there.

4. Transfer the ramekins in the trivet to the pressure cooker and close the lid. Cook at "Steam" mode for 20 minutes.

5. When the dish is cooked, let it rest before serving, which should be done warm.

Nutrition: calories 141, fat 12, fiber 0, carbs 3.5, protein 5.1

Coconut Macaroons

Prep time: 10 minutes

Cooking time: 3 minutes

Servings: 5

Ingredients

- 3 egg whites

- 2 tablespoons Erythritol

- 1 teaspoon vanilla protein powder

- ½ cup almond flour

- ½ cup coconut shred

- 1 teaspoon baking powder

Directions:

1. Whisk the eggs whites in the mixing bowl.

2. Add Erythritol, vanilla protein powder, almond flour, coconut shred, and baking powder. Stir the mixture well.

3. Make the medium size balls from the mixture and press them gently. Place the pressed balls (macaroons) in the Foodie basket.

4. Close the lid and cook on Air fryer mode at 360F for 3 minutes or until thedessert is light brown. Chill little before serving.

Nutrition: calories 118, fat 9.4, fiber 2, carbs 9.3, protein 5.5

Vanilla Bars

Prep time: 10 minutes

Cooking time: 6 minutes

Servings: 8

Ingredients

- 1 cup coconut shred

- 1/3 cup coconut flour

- 2 eggs, whisked

- 3 tablespoons swerve

- 1 teaspoon vanilla extract

- ¼ cup pecans, chopped

- 2 tablespoons butter

Directions:

1. Mix up together coconut shred, coconut flour, whisked eggs, swerve, vanilla extract, and chopped pecans.

2. Then add butter and stir the mass until homogenous. Line the Foodie with baking paper from inside and place coconut mixture on it.

3. Flatten it to get the smooth layer. Close the lid and cook coconut mixture for 6 minutes on High-Pressure mode.

4. Then make quick pressure release. Open the lid and transfer cooked coconut mixture on the plate. Cut it into the serving bars.

Nutrition: calories 182, fat 15.5, fiber 4.4, carbs 13.6, protein 3.4

Avocado and Coconut Mousse

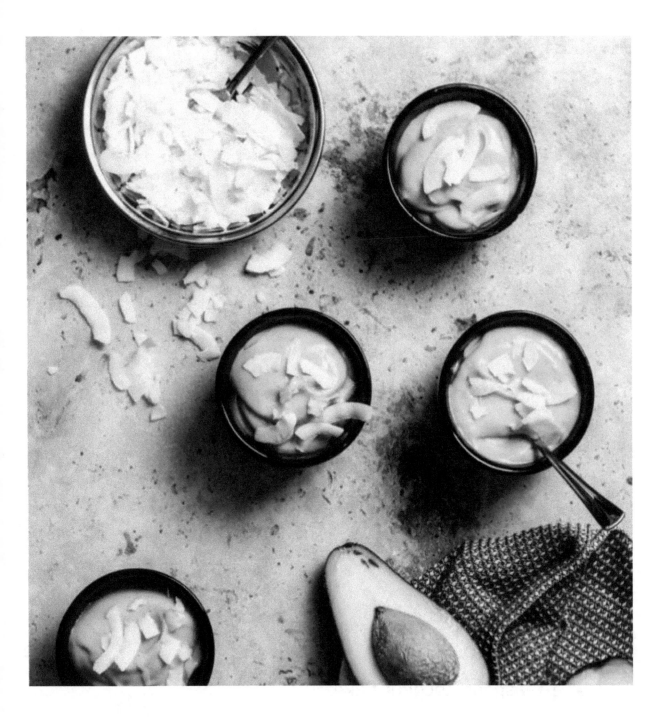

Prep time: 10 minutes

Cooking time: 25 minutes

Servings: 4

Ingredients

- ½ cup almond milk

- 2 egg yolks

- 2 tablespoons swerve

- 2 avocado, peeled

- 1 teaspoon coconut flakes

- 1 teaspoon vanilla extract

Directions:

1. Pour almond milk in the Foodie. Whisk yolks with swerve and vanilla extract. Transfer the mixture in the Foodie.

2. Close the lid and cook on Pressure mode (high pressure) for 3 minutes. Meanwhile, blend the avocado until soft and smooth.

3. Chill the cooked almond milk mixture little. Mix up together blended avocado and almond milk mixture. Stir well.

4. Transfer the dessert into the serving bowls and sprinkle with coconut flakes.

Nutrition: calories 308, fat 29.2, fiber 7.4, carbs 11.8, protein 4

Ricotta and Nutmeg Pie

Prep time: 10 minutes

Cooking time: 20 minutes

Servings: 8

Ingredients

- 14 ounces ricotta cheese

- 4 eggs

- 1/3 cup Erythritol

- 1 cup coconut flour

- 1 teaspoon salt

- 1 tablespoon butter

- 1 teaspoon nutmeg

- 1 tablespoon vanilla extract

- ¼ teaspoon sage

Directions:

1. Whisk the eggs in a mixing bowl and combine it with the ricotta.

2. Stir the mixture and sprinkle it with the salt, nutmeg, Erythritol, vanilla extract, and butter. Mix well and sift the coconut flour into the bowl.

3. Mix the batter until smooth. Pour the batter into the pressure cooker.

4. Flatten it gently using a spatula. Close the lid and cook at "Pressure" mode for 20 minutes.

5. When the cooking time ends, release the pressure and let the pie rest for 10 minutes. Transfer the pie to a serving plate. Slice and serve.

Nutrition: calories 126, fat 7.9, fiber 0.7, carbs 12.1, protein 8.7

Nutmeg Crumble

Prep time: 10 minutes

Cooking time: 25 minutes

Servings: 6

Ingredients

- ⅓ cup Erythritol

- 1 cup almond flour

- 8 ounces butter

- 1 teaspoon cinnamon

- 1 tablespoon nutmeg

- 1 zucchini, chopped

- 1 tablespoon vanilla extract

- ½ cup whipped cream

Directions:

1. Place zucchini in the pressure cooker. Set the pressure cooker to "Sauté" mode. Sprinkle the zucchini with Erythritol and nutmeg.

2. Mix well and sauté it for 10 minutes. Slice the butter.

3. Combine the cinnamon, vanilla extract, and almond flour together. Add the butter and mix well using your hands.

4. Rub the dough using your fingers until a crumbly mixture is achieved. Sprinkle the sautéed zucchini with the crumble dough and close the pressure cooker lid.

5. Cook at "Pressure" mode for 15 minutes.

6. Release the pressure and let the dish rest. Transfer the dish to a serving plate and add whipped cream.

Nutrition: calories 423, fat 43.5, fiber 2.7, carbs 6.1, protein 4.9

Blackberry Compote

Prep time: 8 minutes

Cooking time: 5 minutes

Servings: 5

Ingredients

- 1 ½ cup blackberries

- 3 tablespoons Erythritol

- 1 teaspoon vanilla extract

- ¼ cup of water

Directions:

1. Mash the blackberries gently and place in Foodie.

2. Add Erythritol, vanilla extract, and water. Stir the berries with the help of a wooden spatula. Close the lid and seal it.

3. Cook compote on Pressure mode (High pressure) for 5 minutes. Release the pressure naturally and chill dessert.

Nutrition: calories 21, fat 0.2, fiber 2.3, carbs 11.5, protein 0.6

Sponge Cake

Prep time: 15 minutes

Cooking time: 30minutes

Servings: 8

Ingredients

- 6 eggs

- 2 cups coconut flour

- 1 cup whipped cream

- ½ cup Erythritol

- 1 tablespoon vanilla extract

Directions:

1. Separate the egg yolks and egg whites. Combine the egg yolks with Erythritol and mix well using a hand mixer until fluffy.

2. Whisk the egg whites until you get firm peaks. Sift the coconut flour and vanilla extract into the egg yolk mixture and stir well.

3. Add the egg whites and fold them in gently using a spatula. Add the sponge cake batter to the pressure cooker.

4. Level the batter using the spatula and close the lid. Cook the cake at the "Pressure" mode for 30 minutes.

5. When the dish is cooked, let it rest before serving.

6. Cut the sponge cake in half crossways and spread one part of the sponge cake with the whipped cream.

7. Cover it with the second part of the cake and serve.

Nutrition: calories 111, fat 8.4, fiber 1.3, carbs 2.9, protein 5

Zucchini "Apple" Baked Crisp

Prep time: 10 minutes

Cooking time: 20 minutes

Servings: 6

Ingredients

- 1 pound zucchini

- 2 cups almond flour

- 1/3 cup Erythritol

- 1 tablespoon cinnamon

- 1 teaspoon vanilla extract

- ⅓ teaspoon baking soda

- 7 ounces butter

- 1 cup of water

- ½ cup flax meal

- 11 tablespoon lemon juice

Directions:

1. Chop the zucchini. Place them in the pressure cooker.

2. Combine Erythritol, cinnamon, and 1 cup of the almond flour together. Sprinkle the chopped zucchini with Erythritol mixture.

3. Pour the water over the zucchini mixture.

4. Combine the vanilla extract, the remaining flour, flax meal, baking soda, lemon juice, and butter in a mixing bowl.

5. Combine untilcrumble forms from the mixture.

6. Sprinkle the apple mixture with the crumbles and close the pressure cooker lid.

7. Cook at "Pressure" mode for 20 minutes. When the cooking time ends, let the apple crisp rest before serving.

Nutrition: calories 514, fat 49.2, fiber 8.2, carbs 25.5, protein 11.5

Conclusion

Being an ideal service both for instantaneous pot newbies and skilled split second pot individuals this instant pot cookbook elevates your daily cooking. It makes you look like a professional as well as prepare like a pro. Thanks to the Instant Pot component, this cookbook assists you with preparing simple as well as yummy meals for any kind of budget. Satisfy everybody with hearty suppers, nutritive breakfasts, sweetest treats, and also fun treats. Despite if you cook for one or prepare larger portions-- there's an option for any type of feasible cooking situation. Enhance your techniques on how to prepare in one of the most reliable means utilizing only your split second pot, this recipe book, as well as some persistence to learn quick. Valuable pointers as well as tricks are discreetly included right into every dish to make your family members demand new dishes time and time again. Vegan alternatives, options for meat-eaters and also highly pleasing suggestions to join the whole household at the same table. Eating in your home is a shared experience, and it can be so excellent to satisfy completely at the end of the day. Master your Instant Pot and make the most of this new experience beginning today!

CPSIA information can be obtained
at www.ICGtesting.com
Printed in the USA
BVHW051645140521
607367BV00015B/2041

9 781667 1281